ULTIMATE SUGAR DETOX DIET FOR 50+

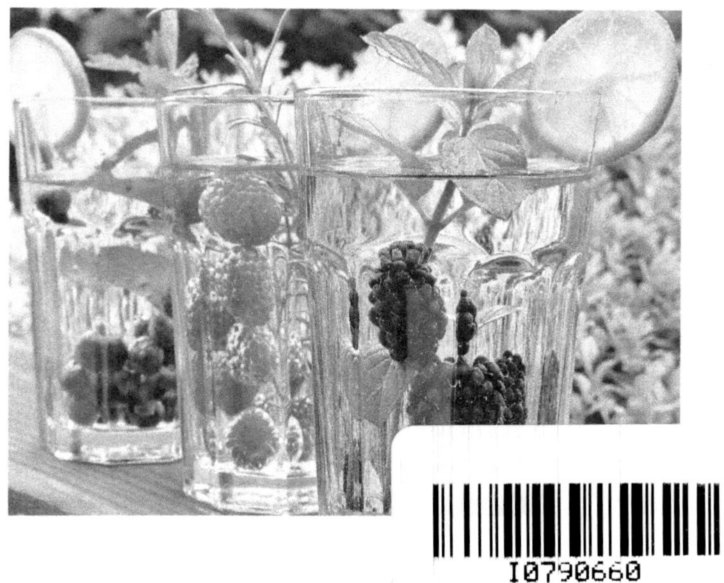

Revitalize Your Health and Reclaim Your Sweet Life

LISA BRITT

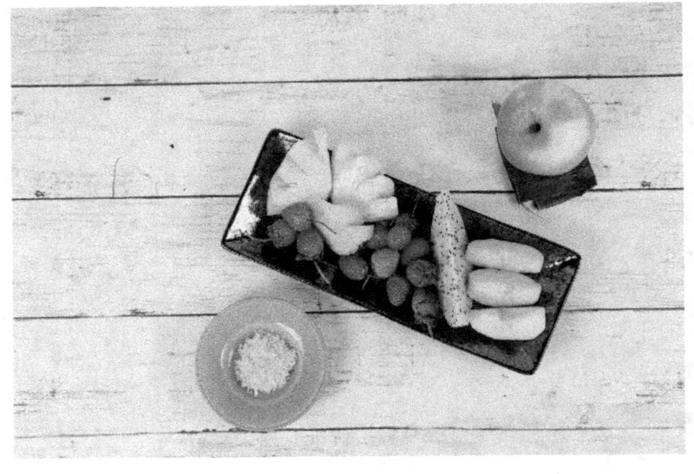

Introduction

Maria, a bright 60-year-old woman, was feeling fatigued and rundown all the time. She had tried everything to feel better, but nothing seemed to work. She opted to see a doctor who did a few tests and discovered that she was pre-diabetic. Her doctor indicated that she needed to make some big changes to her lifestyle, including cutting back on sugar.

Maria was a big admirer of sweets, and the thought of giving them up seemed unthinkable. However, she felt she had to do something to better her health, so she decided to attempt a sugar detox diet for adults over 50. She studied numerous sugar detox diets and found one that appeared fair and sustainable.

Maria started her sugar detox diet by eliminating all sugar from her meals for the first week. She was amazed at how tough it was to cut out sugar totally, but she persevered. During the second and third weeks, she gradually reintroduced a few natural sugars, such as fruits, but avoided processed sugars like the plague.

By the fourth week, Maria felt like a new person. She had more energy, her skin looked better, and her mood was more upbeat. She was happy with the outcomes of the sugar detox diet and wanted to maintain the lifestyle shift. She realized it was not simply a fad diet but a sustainable way of eating that she could maintain long-term.

Maria even started sharing her experience with her friends and family, pushing them to try the sugar detox diet too. She described her new favorite dishes that she discovered, such a delightful sugar-free blueberry smoothie that she now loves every morning.

Maria's road towards a sugar-free diet was not always simple, but she discovered that taking tiny efforts and being consistent can lead to substantial changes. She was grateful for the sugar detox diet that helped her to feel healthier and enjoy life to the fullest. And most significantly, she was delighted that she could continue to enjoy sweets, but now in a better and more aware way.

A.Benefits of a sugar detox for individuals over 50

A sugar detox can be particularly advantageous for persons over 50, as they may be more prone to health issues such as weight gain, high blood pressure, and diabetes. Here are some potential benefits of a sugar detox for those over 50:

Weight loss: As we age, our metabolism slows down, making it tougher to lose weight. Reducing sugar intake can aid with weight loss by reducing calorie consumption and boosting metabolism.

Lowered risk of chronic diseases: A diet heavy in sugar has been associated with an increased risk of chronic diseases such as diabetes, heart disease, and some malignancies. By taking out sugar, adults over 50 can minimize their risk of acquiring these diseases.

Improved cognitive performance: Studies have indicated that a high sugar intake might impair cognitive function, especially in older persons. By limiting sugar intake, adults over 50 can improve their memory and cognitive abilities.

Better oral health: Sugar is a big contributor to tooth damage, and as we age, our teeth become more prone to decay. By limiting sugar intake, adults over 50 can enhance their dental health and reduce the chance of tooth loss.

Improved energy levels: Sugar can create energy dumps and weariness, which can be particularly problematic for older persons. By limiting sugar intake, adults over 50 can boost their energy levels and feel more alert and productive throughout the day.

Overall, a sugar detox can give a number of benefits for persons over 50, including weight loss, enhanced cognitive function, and a lower risk of chronic diseases. However, it's vital to consult a healthcare expert before initiating any big dietary changes, especially if you have any underlying health concerns.

B.Precautions for individuals over 50

The sugar detox diet can be an effective strategy to enhance general health and minimize the risk of chronic diseases such as diabetes, heart disease, and obesity. However, for persons over 50, there are several considerations that should be followed before commencing this diet. Here are some crucial precautions to consider:

Consult with a healthcare provider: Before starting any new diet or fitness program, it is crucial to consult with a healthcare practitioner. This is especially true for persons over 50, who may have pre-existing health concerns that could be harmed by the sugar detox diet.

incremental modifications: Instead of making dramatic changes to your diet, it may be best to make incremental changes over time. This can help prevent any unexpected spikes or fall in blood sugar levels, which can be harmful for persons over 50.

Stay hydrated: It is vital to drink enough water while on the sugar detox diet, especially for persons over 50. Dehydration can be more common in older persons and can lead to major health consequences.

Monitor blood sugar levels: Individuals over 50 who are on the sugar detox diet should monitor their blood sugar levels routinely. This can help prevent any rapid spikes or reductions in blood sugar levels, which can be problematic for persons with pre-existing health issues such as diabetes.

Eat a balanced diet: While the sugar detox diet may limit certain foods, it is crucial to ensure that you are still getting all of the necessary nutrients. Older adults may be at higher risk for nutrient deficiencies, therefore it is vital to consume a balanced diet that includes a range of fruits, vegetables, whole grains, and lean proteins.

Exercise regularly: Regular exercise is vital for persons over 50, since it can assist improve general health and minimize the risk of chronic diseases. However, it is crucial to talk to a healthcare practitioner before starting any new exercise regimen.

monitor for indicators of low blood sugar: Individuals over 50 who are on the sugar detox diet should monitor for signs of low blood sugar, such as dizziness, disorientation, and lethargy. If you experience these symptoms, it is vital to ingest a modest amount of carbs, such as fruit or crackers, to bring your blood sugar levels back up.

In conclusion, the sugar detox diet can be an excellent strategy to enhance overall health and minimize the risk of chronic diseases, however persons over 50 should take measures before starting this diet. It is crucial to speak with a healthcare expert, make moderate changes, remain hydrated, monitor blood sugar levels, eat a balanced diet, exercise regularly, and watch for indicators of low blood sugar.

II. Understanding Sugar and its Effects on the Body

A. What is sugar?

Sugar is a form of carbohydrate that is often used as a sweetener in food and drinks. It is a simple carbohydrate, meaning that it is made up of only one or two sugar molecules. The most prevalent form of sugar is sucrose, which is made up of glucose and fructose molecules. Other forms of sugar include glucose, fructose, lactose, and maltose. Sugar is present naturally in many fruits and vegetables, but it is also often added to processed foods and drinks. While minimal amounts of sugar can be a component of a healthy diet, excessive consumption of sugar has been related to several health concerns, including obesity, diabetes, and tooth decay.

B.How sugar affects the body

Sugar impacts the body in numerous ways. When you take sugar, it is broken down into glucose in the body, which is subsequently absorbed into the bloodstream. The pancreas subsequently releases insulin to assist the body's cells absorb the glucose and utilize it for energy.

However, when you ingest too much sugar, your body may produce too much insulin, which can lead to insulin resistance over time. Insulin resistance is a condition where the cells in the body become less receptive to insulin, making it difficult for the body to use glucose for energy. This can lead to elevated blood sugar levels, which can eventually lead to type 2 diabetes.

In addition to the danger of getting diabetes, ingesting excessive amounts of sugar can also lead to weight gain and obesity. Sugary foods and drinks are generally high in calories, and consuming them might make it difficult to limit calorie consumption, which can contribute to an increase in body weight.

Furthermore, sugar can also lead to tooth decay. Bacteria in the mouth feed on sugar, generating acid that can erode tooth enamel and contribute to cavities.

It is crucial to consume sugar in moderation as part of a balanced diet to avoid these detrimental effects on the body.

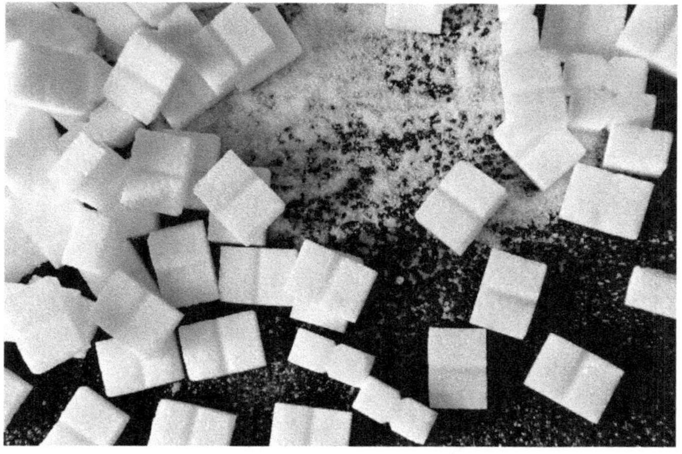

C.Hidden sources of sugar in food

Sugar can be disguised in many processed foods and drinks, even those that may not taste sweet. Here are some common sources of hidden sugar in food:

Condiments and dressings: Many condiments and salad dressings, such as ketchup, barbecue sauce, and ranch dressing, include added sugar.

Beverages: Sugary beverages such as soda, fruit juice, and sports drinks can contain substantial levels of added sugar.

Breakfast cereals: Many breakfast cereals, especially those marketed to children, are rich in added sugar.

Granola bars and energy bars: Many granola and energy bars use additional sugar to improve their taste and texture.

Yogurt: Flavored yogurt can include considerable amounts of added sugar. Choosing plain yogurt and adding fresh fruit can be a healthier alternative.

Baked goods: Cakes, cookies, and pastries generally contain substantial amounts of added sugar.

Processed snacks: Many processed foods, such as chips and crackers, might include added sugar to improve their taste.

Canned and packaged foods: Many canned and packaged goods, such as canned fruit and tomato sauce, might have added sugar.

It's vital to read the ingredients list and nutrition label on packaged foods to identify any added sugars. Choosing whole foods and making meals at home might also help you reduce your sugar intake.

D.The link between sugar and chronic diseases

There is considerable evidence associating excessive consumption of sugar to various chronic conditions, including:

Obesity: Consuming significant amounts of sugar can contribute to weight gain and obesity, which are risk factors for many chronic diseases.

Type 2 diabetes: Excessive consumption of sugar can lead to insulin resistance, which can raise the chance of developing type 2 diabetes.

Cardiovascular disease: High sugar intake has been related to an increased risk of heart disease, stroke, and other cardiovascular disorders.

Non-alcoholic fatty liver disease: Excessive sugar intake can lead to the accumulation of fat in the liver, which can raise the chance of developing non-alcoholic fatty liver disease.

Tooth decay: Consuming significant amounts of sugar might contribute to tooth decay and cavities.

Inflammation: Consuming high levels of sugar can also produce persistent low-grade inflammation, which has been related to various chronic diseases, including cancer, Alzheimer's disease, and arthritis.

Reducing sugar intake can help lessen the chance of acquiring several chronic diseases. It's crucial to consume a balanced diet that includes whole, nutrient-dense foods and minimize intake of processed and sugary meals and drinks.

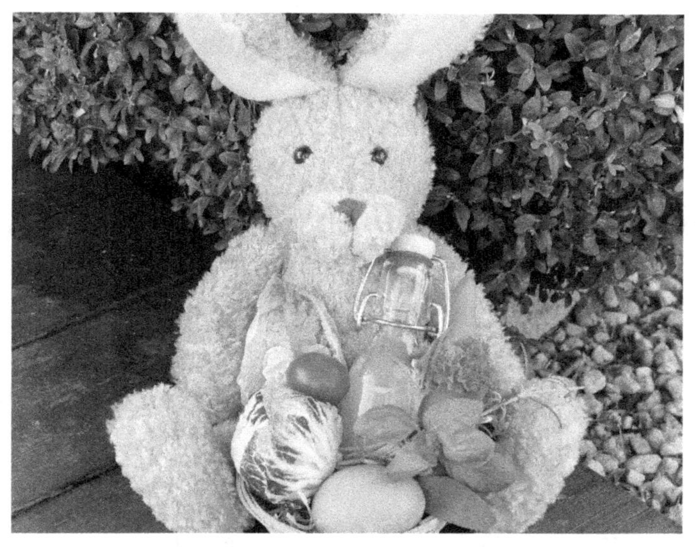

III. Getting Started on the Sugar Detox Diet

A. Preparing for the sugar detox diet

Preparing for a sugar detox diet might be tough, but it is a fantastic method to reset your body and break free from the detrimental consequences of excessive sugar consumption. Sugar detox diets entail removing or substantially limiting your sugar intake for a period of time, often ranging from a few days to a few weeks. Here are some recommendations to help you prepare for a successful sugar detox:

Plan ahead: Before starting the sugar detox diet, take some time to prepare your meals and snacks. Stock up on healthful, whole foods such as veggies, fruits, lean meats, and healthy fats. Make a list of recipes that you can prepare throughout the detox time.

Gradually reduce your sugar intake: It can be difficult to eliminate sugar from your diet cold turkey. Instead, gradually lower your sugar intake in the days preceding up to the detox. This can help lessen the symptoms of sugar withdrawal.

Stay hydrated: Drinking plenty of water is vital during a sugar detox. Water helps wash away pollutants and keeps you hydrated. Aim to drink at least 8-10 glasses of water per day.

Get lots of rest: During the first few days of the sugar detox, you may experience lethargy and other symptoms as your body adjusts to the new diet. Getting enough rest might help your body cope with these changes.

Avoid processed foods: Processed foods are often filled with sugar and can ruin your sugar detox attempts. Instead, choose for entire, nutrient-dense foods that will nourish your body and keep you feeling full.

Find healthy alternatives to sugar: There are plenty of healthy alternatives to sugar that you can take during the detox period, such as stevia, monk fruit, or honey. These can help satisfy your sweet desire without adding extra sugar to your diet.

Stay motivated: Finally, remember why you are doing the sugar detox and stay motivated. Focus on the benefits you will experience, such as greater energy levels, better sleep, and clearer skin. Celebrate your progress along the way and don't give up if you slip up.

In conclusion, preparing for a sugar detox diet involves forethought, discipline, and commitment. With these guidelines, you can set yourself up for success and realize the benefits of a healthier, sugar-free lifestyle.

B.Planning meals and snacks

Planning meals and snacks for a sugar detox diet is a vital aspect of a successful detox. It might be tough to find dishes that are both gratifying and free of added sugars, but with a little imagination, it's possible to come up with delicious and healthy meal options. Here are some recommendations for organizing meals and snacks for a sugar detox diet:

Focus on entire foods: When preparing meals and snacks, focus on whole foods such as fruits, vegetables, lean meats, and healthy fats. These foods will offer your body with the nutrition it needs while keeping you full and content.

Incorporate healthy fats: Healthy fats, such as avocado, almonds, and olive oil, will help keep you feeling full and pleased while also giving your body with critical nutrients. Incorporate these healthy fats into your meals and snacks to help balance your blood sugar levels and prevent cravings.

Use natural sweeteners: While it's crucial to avoid additional sugars throughout the detox period, you can still use natural sweeteners such as stevia, monk fruit, or honey in moderation. These sweeteners can help satisfy your sweet taste without increasing your blood sugar levels.

Plan ahead: Take some time to plan your meals and snacks for the week ahead. This might help you avoid impulse purchases and ensure that you have healthy options on hand when cravings occur.

Mix and match: Don't be scared to mix and match different foods to make fulfilling and delicious meals and snacks. For example, you may construct a smoothie bowl using Greek yogurt, berries, and chia seeds

C.Tips for grocery shopping

If you're on a sugar detox diet, grocery shopping can be a bit hard. It's crucial to choose the correct foods to support your health and avoid those that could derail your progress. Here are some pointers to help you make the most of your next grocery shopping trip:

Stick to the perimeter of the store: Most grocery stores have their produce, meats, and dairy areas on the outer corners of the store. These are the regions where you'll discover the freshest, least processed goods. Try to focus your purchasing on these areas, and avoid the central aisles, where most of the processed items are situated.

Look for entire foods: When shopping for a sugar detox diet, focus on whole, natural foods. Fresh fruits and vegetables, lean proteins, nuts, and seeds should make up the bulk of your shopping cart. Avoid processed foods like chips, cookies, and other snacks, which are generally filled with added sugars.

Read labels carefully: Sugar is added to many processed foods, including ones that don't taste sweet. When shopping, make sure to read the labels carefully and check for added sugars under any of the following names: sucrose, fructose, glucose, maltose, dextrose, and high-fructose corn syrup. Avoid items that contain sugar or any of these components high up on the ingredient list.

Choose low-glycemic options: Foods with a high glycemic index, such as white bread, potatoes, and candies, can induce a quick jump in blood sugar levels. Instead, opt for foods with a low glycemic index, such as leafy greens, berries, and whole grains. These foods release glucose into the bloodstream more slowly, helping to keep your blood sugar levels constant.

Plan ahead: Before heading to the grocery shop, make a list of the goods you need and plan out your meals for the week. This can help you avoid impulse buys and ensure that you have lots of healthy, sugar-free options on hand when hunger strikes.

In essence, food shopping for a sugar detox diet demands careful planning and attention to detail. By focusing on whole, natural foods, reading labels carefully, and choosing low-glycemic options, you can set yourself up for success and make the most of   your   sugar   detox   diet.

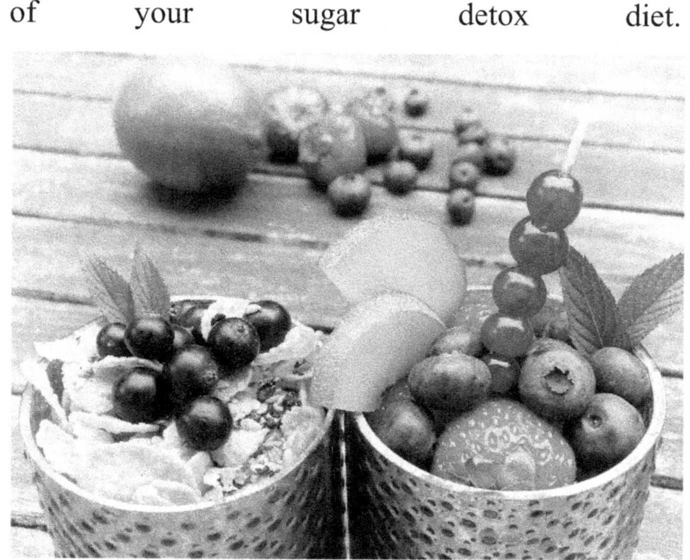

IV. The Sugar Detox Diet Meal Plan

A.Week 1: Elimination Phase

Congratulations for taking the first step towards a healthy lifestyle by going on a sugar detox diet! The elimination phase of this diet can be unpleasant, but it's vital to stay with it to reap the benefits in the long run.

During the first week of the elimination phase, your goal is to eliminate all kinds of sugar from your diet. This includes industrial sugar, artificial sweeteners, and even natural sugars found in fruits and honey. By eliminating sugar from your diet, you'll be giving your body an opportunity to reset and break free from its need for sugar.

Here's a sample meal plan for the first week of the elimination phase:

Breakfast:

Scrambled eggs with spinach and mushroomsAvocado slicesUnsweetened almond milk

Lunch:

Grilled chicken breastMixed greens salad with cucumbers and cherry tomatoesOlive oil and balsamic vinegar dressing

Snack:

Raw vegetables with hummus

Dinner:

Baked salmonRoasted broccoli and cauliflowerQuinoa

It's crucial to drink enough water throughout the day and to respond to your body's hunger cues. If you're feeling hungry between meals, go for nutritious snacks like raw vegetables with hummus or a handful of nuts.

Remember, the first week of the elimination phase can be rough, but it's worth it to break free from your dependence on sugar. Stick with it, and you'll start to feel the advantages in no time!

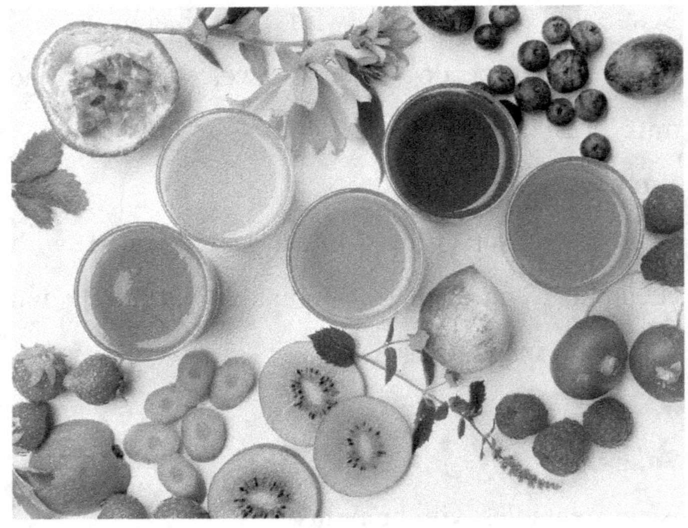

B.Week 2-3: Transition Phase

The transition phase of a sugar detox diet meal plan often happens during weeks 2 and 3 of the program. This is a vital stage where your body is adjusting to the new diet and trying to cope with the absence of sugar.

During this phase, it is vital to avoid all forms of added sugars, including white sugar, brown sugar, high fructose corn syrup, honey, agave nectar, and maple syrup. You should also avoid all processed foods, which typically include hidden sugars.

Instead, focus on eating entire meals that are high in fiber, protein, healthy fats, and complex carbohydrates. Some good options are vegetables, fruits, whole grains, nuts, seeds, and lean proteins like chicken, fish, and tofu.

To assist you make the move simpler, here are some tips:

Stay hydrated: Drinking plenty of water will help flush out toxins and keep you feeling full and pleased.

Eat frequent, little meals: Instead of three large meals a day, try eating five or six smaller meals to keep your blood sugar levels steady.

Be prepared: Plan your meals in advance and make sure you have healthy snacks on hand to prevent reaching for sugary munchies.

Focus on healthy fats: Incorporate healthy fats like avocado, almonds, and olive oil into your meals to help you feel full and content.

Use natural sweeteners: If you need a little sweetness in your food, try using natural sweeteners like stevia or monk fruit.

Be patient: It can take time for your body to acclimate to the new diet, so be patient and stick with it.

Remember, the transition phase is a vital moment in your sugar detox journey. By following these recommendations and keeping committed to your new lifestyle, you will be on your road to a healthier, happier self.

C.Week 4: Reintroduction Phase

The Reintroduction Phase is the fourth week of the sugar detox diet meal plan. During this phase, you will slowly reintroduce some foods back into your diet to evaluate how your body responds. This can help you understand which foods are triggers for your sugar cravings and which ones you can accept in moderation.

Here are some tips to follow during the Reintroduction Phase:

Start Slow: Start by introducing one new food group at a time. For example, if you want to reintroduce dairy, start with a little amount of plain yogurt or cheese.

Monitor Your Body: Pay special attention to how your body reacts to the reintroduced food. If you suffer any unpleasant effects like bloating, headaches, or exhaustion, you may need to omit that food group from your diet for a longer period of time.

Choose entire Foods: Stick to entire, nutrient-dense foods and avoid processed foods or added sweets.

Keep a Food Journal: Write down what you eat and how you feel after eating it. This will help you track which foods provoke cravings or bad feelings.

Be Mindful of Portions: Just because you're reintroducing a food category doesn't imply you can eat endless amounts of it. Be cautious of portion sizes and listen to your body's hunger cues.

Some things you can consider reintroducing during this phase include:

Whole grains such as quinoa, brown rice, or oats.

Dairy goods such as basic yogurt, cheese, or milk.

Fruits having a low glycemic index such as berries or apples.

Natural sweeteners such as honey or maple syrup (in modest doses).

Remember, the purpose of the Reintroduction Phase is to establish which foods work for your body and which ones don't. Be patient with the process and be open to modifying your diet as needed. By the end of this phase, you should have a better grasp of how to maintain a balanced and healthy diet while regulating your sugar cravings.

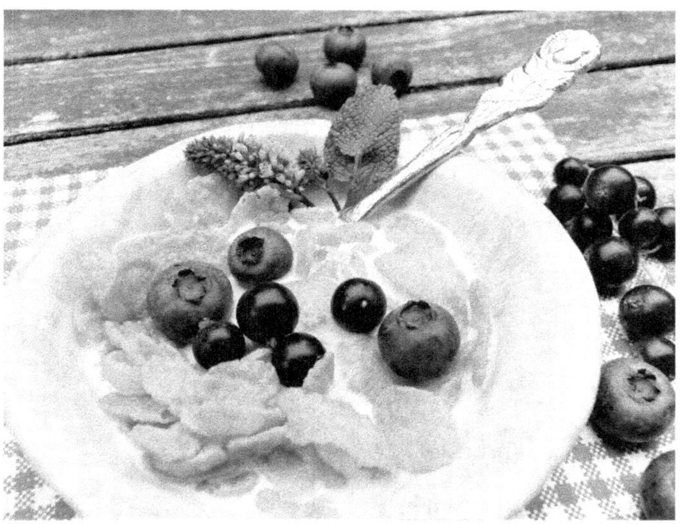

V. Sugar Detox Diet Recipes for Individuals Over 50

A.Breakfast recipes

Avocado with Egg Breakfast Bowl: Mash half an avocado and mix it with a scrambled egg. Serve with sliced cherry tomatoes, spinach leaves, and a sprinkle of salt and pepper.

Chia Seed Pudding: Mix 1/4 cup of chia seeds with 1 cup of unsweetened almond milk and let it sit in the fridge overnight. In the morning, top with sliced fruit and nuts.

Greek Yogurt with Berries: Top a small dish of plain Greek yogurt with a handful of fresh berries and a drizzle of honey or a sprinkle of cinnamon.

Veggie Omelet: Whisk 2 eggs with a dash of unsweetened almond milk. Cook in a non-stick pan with sliced bell peppers, onions, and mushrooms. Serve with a side of sliced avocado.

Sweet Potato Hash: Grate 1 small sweet potato and sauté in a non-stick pan with sliced onions and a handful of spinach. Top with a fried egg and a sprinkling of paprika.

Remember to avoid adding any sweeteners, including honey or maple syrup, since these can disrupt your sugar detox attempts. Instead, focus on using fresh, whole ingredients to produce great and satisfying breakfasts. And as always, contact your healthcare physician before making any big dietary changes.

B.Lunch recipes

Chicken and vegetable stir-fry: This meal is filled with protein and nutritious vegetables. Start by stir-frying cubed chicken breast in coconut oil. Add chopped vegetables like broccoli, bell peppers, and onions, and continue to stir-fry until the vegetables are soft. Season with herbs and spices like garlic, ginger, and cumin for extra flavor.

Quinoa salad: Quinoa is a high-protein grain that's great for a sugar detox diet. Cook quinoa according to package instructions and mix it with diced vegetables like cucumber, cherry tomatoes, and bell peppers. Dress the salad with a simple vinaigrette made with olive oil, lemon juice, and Dijon mustard.

Sweet potato and black bean burrito bowl: This recipe is a terrific way to fulfill a taste for Mexican food without all the additional sugar. Start by cooking chopped sweet potato in the oven with a little bit of olive oil and salt. Then, combine cooked black beans with corn, sliced tomatoes, and cilantro. Serve the mixture over brown rice and top with the roasted sweet potato and a dollop of Greek yogurt.

Salmon and veggie kebabs: These kebabs are a terrific way to get in some healthful omega-3 fatty acids. Cut salmon into slices and skewer it with vegetables like cherry tomatoes, zucchini, and red onion. Brush the kebabs with a mixture of olive oil, lemon juice, and herbs like thyme and oregano before grilling.

Lentil soup: Lentils are an excellent source of plant-based protein and fiber, making them an ideal complement to a sugar detox diet. Cook lentils in vegetable broth with chopped veggies like carrots, celery, and onion. Add herbs and spices like cumin, coriander, and turmeric for extra flavor.

Remember to read food labels carefully and avoid added sugars in processed foods when following a sugar detox diet. Enjoy your lunch!

C.Dinner recipes

Here are three dinner ideas for a sugar detox diet that are suited for adults over 50:

Baked Salmon with Roasted Vegetables Ingredients:

4 salmon filets

2 medium-sized zucchinis, sliced 1 large red bell pepper, sliced 1 large yellow onion, sliced 2 cloves garlic, minced 1 tbsp olive oil

Salt and pepper to taste

Instructions:

Preheat the oven to 400°F.

In a large bowl, add sliced zucchini, red bell pepper, onion, garlic, olive oil, salt, and pepper. Mix well.

Line a baking sheet with parchment paper and distribute the veggie mixture on the sheet.

Bake in the preheated oven for 20 minutes, stirring occasionally.

Season the salmon filets with salt and pepper and arrange them on top of the roasted veggies.

Bake for a further 10-15 minutes or until the salmon is cooked through.

Turkey Chili

Ingredients:

1 pound ground turkey

1 large onion, chopped 2 garlic cloves, minced 1 red bell pepper, chopped 1 green bell pepper, chopped 1 can (14.5 oz) chopped tomatoes

1 can (15 oz) kidney beans, drained and rinsed

2 tbsp chili powder

1 tsp cumin

1 tsp oregano

Salt and pepper to taste

Instructions:

Heat a big pot over medium heat.

Add ground turkey and heat until browned.

Add chopped onion and garlic, and sauté until the onion is tender.

Add chopped red and green bell pepper and simmer for 5 minutes.

Add diced tomatoes, kidney beans, chili powder, cumin, oregano, salt, and pepper. Stir thoroughly.

Simmer the chili for 30 minutes, stirring occasionally.

Baked Chicken with Roasted Broccoli

Ingredients:

4 chicken breasts

1 pound broccoli florets

2 garlic cloves, minced

1 tbsp olive oil

Salt and pepper to taste

Instructions:

Preheat the oven to 400°F.

Line a baking sheet with parchment paper.

In a large bowl, mix broccoli florets, minced garlic, olive oil, salt, and pepper. Toss well to coat.

Spread the broccoli mixture on the baking sheet.

Place the chicken breasts on top of the broccoli.

Bake for 25-30 minutes or until the chicken is cooked through.

These dinner recipes are tasty, healthful, and suitable for persons over 50 who want to follow a sugar detox diet. They are low in sugar, high in protein, and full of healthful vegetables. Enjoy!

D.Snack recipes

Sugar detox diets can be tough, especially for persons over 50 who may have developed a stronger taste for sweets over the years. However, there are many delicious snack options that can help fulfill your cravings and keep you on track with your sugar detox goals. Here are some snack recipes for sugar detox diets that are excellent for folks over 50:

Apple slices with almond butter: Cut up an apple into thin slices and serve with a tablespoon of almond butter. Almond butter is a terrific source of healthy fats and protein, and the sweetness of the apple will help curb your sugar cravings.

Roasted chickpeas: Drain and rinse a can of chickpeas and combine with a tablespoon of olive oil and your favorite spices, such as garlic powder, cumin, and paprika. Roast in the oven at 400°F for 20-25 minutes, or until crispy. Chickpeas are an excellent source of fiber and protein, and the spices will add taste without any added sugar.

Greek yogurt with berries: Mix a serving of Greek yogurt with a handful of fresh berries, such as strawberries, blueberries, or raspberries. Greek yogurt is high in protein and low in sugar, and the natural sweetness of the berries can help satisfy your sweet taste.

Hard-boiled eggs: Hard-boiled eggs are a quick and easy snack that are strong in protein and low in sugar. Add a sprinkling of salt and pepper for flavor.

Carrot sticks with hummus: Cut up some carrots into sticks and serve with a tablespoon of hummus. Hummus is a terrific source of protein and healthy fats, and the crunch of the carrots can help satisfy your needs for something crispy.

Kale chips: Remove the stems from a bunch of kale and shred the leaves into bite-sized pieces. Toss with a tablespoon of olive oil and a sprinkle of salt, then bake in the oven at 350°F for 10-15 minutes, or until crispy. Kale is an excellent source of fiber and vitamins, and the chips make a great low-sugar snack.

Avocado toast: Mash half an avocado and spread it across a slice of whole-grain bread. Top with a sprinkle of salt and pepper, and maybe a squeeze of lemon juice. Avocado is high in healthful fats and fiber, and the bread gives a pleasant crunch.

These sugar detox snack recipes for those over 50 are not only delicious but also nutritious and will help you remain on track with your sugar detox goals

E.Dessert recipes

If you're over 50 and following a sugar detox diet, you may be wondering if you may still eat desserts. The good news is that there are many delicious and healthful dessert options that don't rely on sugar. Here are three dessert dishes that are great for anyone following a sugar detox diet.

Berry Coconut Yogurt Parfait Ingredients:

1 cup full-fat coconut yogurt

1 cup mixed berries (strawberries, blueberries, raspberries)

1/4 cup unsweetened shredded coconut

Instructions:

In a small bowl, mix together the coconut yogurt and shredded coconut.

In a second bowl, mash half of the mixed berries with a fork to release their juices.

In a small glass, layer the coconut yogurt mixture, mashed berries, and whole berries until the glass is filled.

Top with extra shredded coconut, if desired, and serve.

Chocolate Chia Pudding

Ingredients:

1/4 cup chia seeds

1 cup unsweetened almond milk

1/4 cup cocoa powder

1 tsp vanilla extract

1 tbsp pure maple syrup (optional)

Fresh berries, for serving

Instructions:

In a large dish, whisk together the chia seeds, almond milk, chocolate powder, vanilla extract, and maple syrup (if using).

Cover the bowl and refrigerate for at least 2 hours or overnight, until the mixture thickens and the chia seeds absorb the liquid.

Serve the chocolate chia pudding topped with fresh berries.

Baked Apples with Cinnamon and Walnuts

Ingredients:

2 apples, cored and sliced into thin rings

1 tsp cinnamon

1/4 cup chopped walnuts

2 tbsp coconut oil, melted

Instructions:

Preheat the oven to 350°F.

In a large bowl, combine together the apple slices, cinnamon, and chopped walnuts.

Drizzle the melted coconut oil over the mixture and toss again to coat.

Spread the apple mixture in a single layer on a baking sheet fitted with parchment paper.

Bake for 20-25 minutes, until the apples are soft and the walnuts are toasted.

Serve the baked apples warm, topped with more chopped walnuts if preferred.

These dessert dishes are a terrific way to fulfill your sweet appetite while following a sugar detox diet. They're packed with nutritional components like berries, coconut, chia seeds, and almonds, and they're free from refined sugars. Enjoy!

VI. Maintaining a Sugar-Free Lifestyle After the Detox

A.Tips for maintaining a sugar-free lifestyle

Maintaining a sugar-free lifestyle can be tough, but it is well worth it for the health benefits. Here are some recommendations to help you stay to a sugar-free lifestyle:

Read labels: Be conscious of the ingredients in the food and drinks you eat. Many foods have hidden sugars, therefore it is vital to read labels carefully.

Avoid processed foods: Processed foods generally have additional sugars, so it's best to stick to full, natural foods like fruits, vegetables, whole grains, and lean meats.

Plan your meals: Plan your meals and snacks ahead of time to avoid the temptation of reaching for a sugary snack when you're hungry and in a rush.

Find healthier alternatives: There are several natural sweeteners that can be used as an alternative to sugar such as stevia, monk fruit, and xylitol. Try using them in your cooking and baking to fulfill your sweet taste.

Drink plenty of water: Drinking water can help suppress cravings and keep you hydrated.

obtain enough sleep: Lack of sleep can contribute to increased desires for sweets, thus it is crucial to obtain enough sleep every night.

Find support: Join a support group or find a buddy who is also attempting to maintain a sugar-free diet. Having a support system can help keep you motivated and accountable.

Remember that making lifestyle changes requires time and effort. Be patient with yourself and enjoy minor triumphs along the road.

B.Strategies for dealing with sugar cravings

Sugar cravings can be tricky to deal with, especially if you're attempting to maintain a sugar-free lifestyle. Here are some ways that may help you manage sugar cravings:

Drink water: Sometimes we mistake thirst for hunger or sugar cravings. Try drinking a glass of water when you sense a craving coming on to see if it helps.

Eat protein and fiber-rich foods: Protein and fiber help you feel full and satisfied, minimizing the probability of sugar cravings. Snack on nuts, seeds, and fruits to help reduce cravings.

Find healthy alternatives: Look for healthier alternatives to sugary indulgences, such as fresh fruits, yogurt, or sugar-free snacks. This can help satisfy your sweet appetite without compromising your sugar-free lifestyle.

Practice mindful eating: Be present and attentive when you eat. Take your time, savor your food, and pay attention to how it makes you feel.

Get moving: Exercise releases endorphins, which can help reduce stress and sugar cravings. Try going for a stroll, doing yoga, or engaging in any other physical activity you enjoy.

Manage stress: Stress can drive sugar cravings, so it's vital to find healthy ways to manage it. Practice relaxing techniques such as meditation, deep breathing, or taking a warm bath.

Get adequate sleep: Lack of sleep can induce sugar cravings, thus it is necessary to get enough rest. Aim for 7-9 hours of sleep each night.

Remember, sugar cravings are natural, and it's alright to indulge occasionally. However, if you're aiming to maintain a sugar-free lifestyle, it's crucial to be careful of your choices and keep on track.

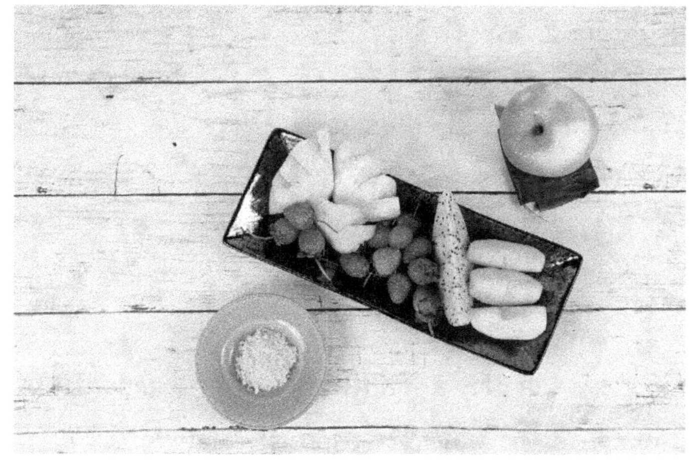

VII. Exercise and Sugar Detox

A.The role of exercise in a sugar detox

Exercise can play a significant role in a sugar detox. Here are some ways that exercise can help:

Reduces stress: Exercise is a great stress-reliever, and stress can trigger sugar cravings. By reducing stress, you may be less likely to reach for sugary treats.

Increases endorphins: Exercise releases endorphins, which are natural mood-boosters. This can help reduce feelings of anxiety and depression, which can contribute to sugar cravings.

Improves insulin sensitivity: Regular exercise can help improve insulin sensitivity, which is important for regulating blood sugar levels. This can reduce sugar cravings and help prevent conditions like diabetes.

Boosts metabolism: Exercise can help boost your metabolism, which can help you burn more calories throughout the day. This can help you maintain a healthy weight, which can also help reduce sugar cravings.

Promotes better sleep: Regular exercise can help improve sleep quality, which can help reduce sugar cravings. Poor sleep can cause hormonal imbalances that can lead to increased appetite and sugar cravings.

Provides distraction: When you're exercising, you're focused on the activity at hand, which can help distract you from sugar cravings.

It's important to note that exercise alone may not be enough to overcome sugar cravings. A comprehensive sugar detox plan should also include healthy eating habits, stress management techniques, and a support system.

B.Recommended exercises for individuals over 50

There are many exercises that can be beneficial for individuals over 50. Here are some recommended exercises:

Walking: Walking is a low-impact exercise that can improve cardiovascular health, strengthen bones and muscles, and improve mood.

Strength training: Strength training can help build and maintain muscle mass, which can help reduce the risk of falls and injuries. Exercises such as squats, lunges, and push-ups can be effective.

Yoga: Yoga can help improve flexibility, balance, and posture, which can help reduce the risk of falls. It can also be a great stress-reliever.

Swimming: Swimming is a low-impact exercise that can be gentle on joints while still providing a good cardiovascular workout.

Cycling: Cycling is a great way to improve cardiovascular health and leg strength. It can also be a low-impact exercise if done on a stationary bike.

Pilates: Pilates can help improve core strength, flexibility, and balance, which can help reduce the risk of falls.

Tai Chi: Tai Chi is a gentle, low-impact exercise that can improve balance, flexibility, and reduce stress.

It's important to start slowly and gradually increase intensity and duration. It's also important to consult with a healthcare provider before starting a new exercise program, especially if you have any underlying health conditions.

VIII. Conclusion

In conclusion, the sugar detox diet for adults over 50 can be a beautiful and beneficial decision for both their short-term and long-term health. By eliminating excess sugar from their diet, individuals can experience a number of benefits such as improved blood sugar control, lower risk of chronic diseases such as diabetes and heart disease, and enhanced cognitive performance.

Furthermore, the sugar detox diet can lead to weight loss and enhanced energy levels, helping individuals to feel more confident and productive in their daily life. Additionally, the diet promotes the consumption of nutrient-rich whole foods, such as fruits, vegetables, lean proteins, and healthy fats, which can assist in satisfying the special nutritional demands of older persons.

Incorporating regular exercise and stress management skills alongside the sugar detox diet might further boost its advantages and promote general well-being. With careful planning and preparation, the sugar detox diet may be both enjoyable and sustainable, making it a profitable investment in one's health and pleasure.

Overall, the sugar detox diet can be a helpful tool for adults over 50 to enhance their health and quality of life. By prioritizing nutritious foods, exercise, and stress management, individuals can experience the benefits of this diet for years to come.